Innovative & Tasty Mediterranean Sea Cookbook

Eat Better with These Mediterranean Recipes

Mateo Buscema

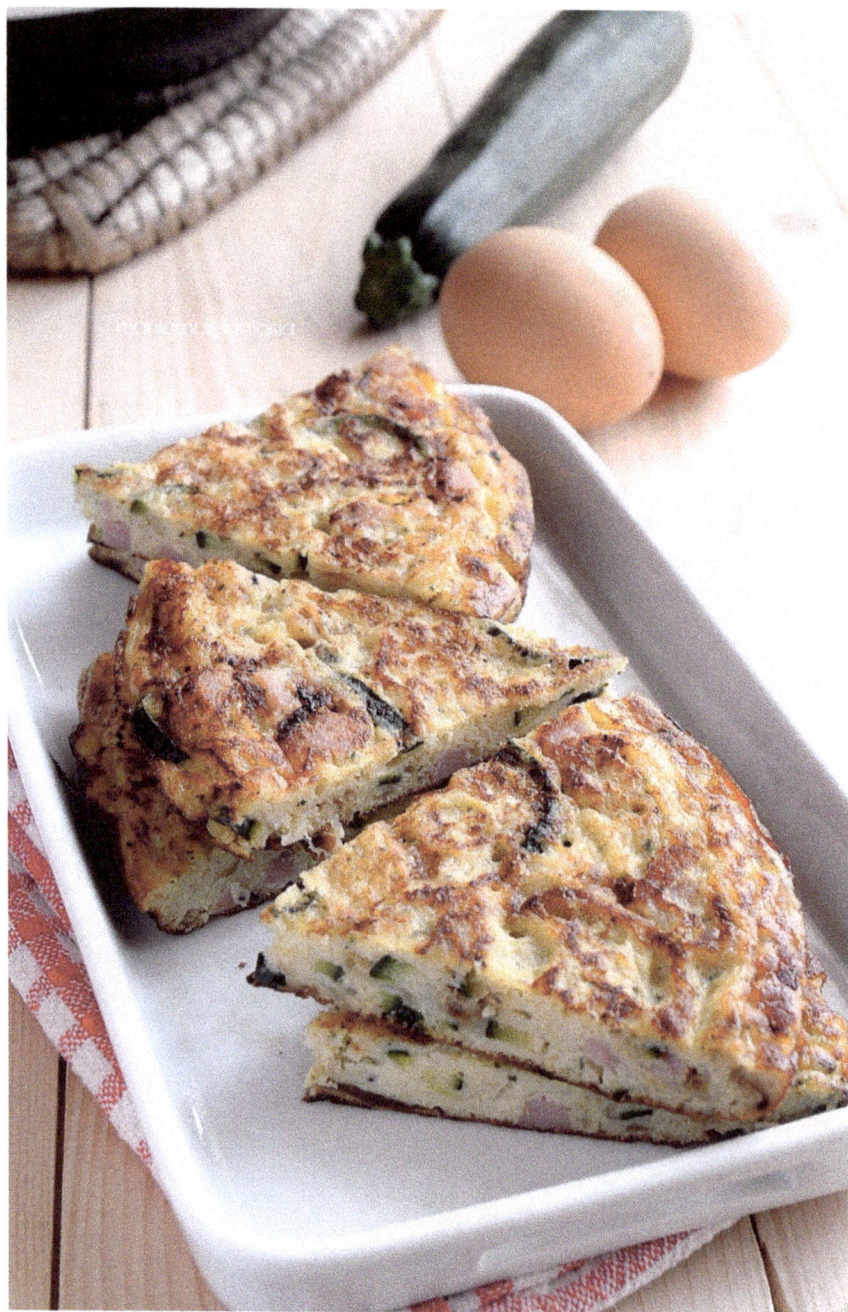

TABLE OF CONTENTS

MEDITERRANEAN STYLE BEAN DIP WITH ROASTED SQUASH................................7

EGYPTIAN KOSHARI RECIPE 9

MEDITERRANEAN PAN SEARED SEA BASS RECIPE WITH A GARLIC BELL PEPPER

MEDLEY 12

PERSIAN BAKED OMELET 15

LENTIL BOLOGNESE SAUCE 17

HOMEMADE VEGETABLE LASAGNA 19

BROCCOLI CURRY 22

CAULIFLOWER CHICKEN CURRY 25

TUNA BURRITO..27

CREAMY TUNA PASTA BAKE 29

PRESSURE CRANBERRY CHICKEN 31

PRESSURE POT PASTA WITH MUSHROOM AND SPINACH................................33

ZUCCHINI LASAGNA..35

PRESSURE POT ZUCCHINI MUSHROOM RISOTTO 38

MEDITERRANEAN GRILLED VEGETABLES 40

ASH ROASTED POTATOES 42

EASY CAMPFIRE POTATOES 43

BUFFALO CHICKEN TACOS 45

EASY SHEPHERD'S PIE...47

SWEET POTATO GNOCCHI 49

CORNED BEEF MASHED POTATOES...51

LENTIL CURRY RECIPE 53

VIETNAMESE SANDWICH BANH MI..55

PRESSURE POT STUFFED TOMATOES 57

PRESSURE POT STUFFED WITH SWEET POTATOES 59

CABBAGE AND SAUSAGE FOIL PACKETS......................................61

SKILLET CHICKEN FAJITAS..63

SPINACH AND ASPARAGUS FRITTATA.......................................65

SPINACH AND CHEDDAR QUICHE..67

ARTICHOKE TART...70

CHILAQUILES VERDE WITH BAKED TORTILLA CHIPS 72

VEGAN MAC AND CHEESE..74

ALMOND SESAME SODA NOODLES WITH QUICK-PICKLED VEGGIES.....76

BROCCOLINI ALMOND PIZZA 78

HUMMUS QUESADILLAS...80

LENTIL BAKED ZITI..81

SPRING VEGGIE STIR FRY 83

SWEET POTATO AND BLACK BEAN TACOS 85

VEGAN BLT SANDWICH...88

VEGAN SPAGHETTI ALLA PUTTANESCA 90

ZUCCHINI NOODLES WITH BASIL PUMPKIN 92

BETTER BROCCOLI CASSEROLE...93

SPINACH PASTA WITH ROASTED BROCCOLI AND BELL PEPPER............................95

SPAGHETTI SQUASH BURRITO BOWLS...97

PASTA PRIMAVERA 99

LEMON BROCCOLI PESTO PASTA 101

STUFFED TOMATO RECIPE 103

CLASSIC TIRAMISU..106

ZA'ATAR MANAQUISH RECIPE 109

Mediterranean style bean dip with roasted squash

Ingredients

- Extra virgin olive oil
- ¾ teaspoon of ground coriander
- 2 tablespoons of toasted pine nuts for garnish
- 2 shallots, peeled and thinly sliced
- ¾ teaspoon of ground cumin
- 2 tablespoons of toasted slivered almonds
- 2 teaspoon of fresh lemon juice
- 1 15-oz. can of cannellini beans, drained and rinsed
- 1 garlic clove, chopped
- ¾ teaspoon of Spanish paprika
- 1 Acorn squash
- ½ teaspoon of cayenne pepper
- Flat leaf parsley for garnish
- ¾ teaspoon of ground sumac

Directions

1. Start by preheating your oven to 400°F.

2. Place acorn squash in microwave and heat on high for 3 minutes.
3. Cut the acorn squash in half through the stem.
4. Scoop out the seeds using a spoon.
5. Sprinkle the squash with salt, put them flesh side down on a lightly oiled baking sheet.
6. Roast in the preheated oven for 40 minutes until flesh is tender and slightly browned.
7. In a skillet, heat 1 tablespoon of extra virgin olive oil over medium-high.
8. Add the shallots and let sauté until caramelized, keep tossing regularly.
9. Season with salt.
10. Remove squash from the oven let cool down.
11. Scoop out the flesh and discard shell.
12. In the bowl of a large food processor, add ½ amount of shallots, squash, white beans, all the spices and then sprinkle with a pinch of salt.
13. Add lemon juice and 3 tablespoon of extra virgin olive oil.
14. Then, close the top of your processor let blend until desired a smooth dip.
15. Taste and adjust accordingly.
16. Shift the dip to a serving bowl.
17. Add a drizzle of olive oil together with the parsley leaves and toasted nuts.
18. Serve and enjoy with warm pita.

Egyptian koshari recipe

Egyptian koshari recipe as the name suggests, it is a typical Egyptian Mediterranean recipe with variety of vegetables especially, onions, tomatoes, garlic for tasty aromatic flavor.

Ingredients

- ½ teaspoon of crushed red pepper flakes
- 1 can of 28-oz. tomato sauce
- ⅓ cup of all-purpose flour
- ½ cup of cooking oil
- 1 teaspoon of ground coriander
- Cooking oil
- 1 small onion, grated
- 1 large onion, sliced into thin rings
- 2 tablespoons of distilled white vinegar
- 4 garlic cloves, minced
- Salt and pepper
- Salt

For Koshari

- 1 15-oz. can of chickpeas, rinsed, drained and warmed
- Water
- ½ teaspoon of each salt and pepper

- ½ teaspoon of coriander
- 1 ½ cup brown lentils, picked over and well-rinsed
- Cooking oil
- 1 ½ cup medium-grain rice, rinsed, soaked
- 2 cups of elbow pasta

Directions

1. Sprinkle the onion rings with salt, then toss them in the flour to coat. Shake off any excess flour.
2. In a large skillet, heat cooking oil over medium heat, cook the onion rings, stirring often, until caramelized brown within 18 minutes.
3. In a saucepan, heat 1 tablespoon of cooking oil.
4. Add the grated onion, cook on medium until the onion turns a translucent.
5. Add the garlic together with the coriander, and red pepper flakes, then sauté until fragrant in 45 seconds.
6. Stir in tomato sauce and pinch of salt.
7. Let simmer over low heat until the sauce thickens in 15 minutes.
8. Stir in the distilled white vinegar, and turn the heat to low.
9. Cover and keep warm.
10. Bring lentils to boil with 4 cups of water in a medium pot over high heat.

11. Lower the heat let continue to cook until lentils are just tender.

12. Drain any excess water.

13. Season with a little salt.

14. Drain the rice from its soaking water.

15. Combine the par-cooked lentils and the rice in the saucepan over medium heat with 1 tablespoon of cooking oil, salt, pepper, and coriander.

16. For 3 minutes, let cook while stirring regularly.

17. Add warm water to cover the rice and lentil mixture.

18. Bring to a boil let the water reduce a little.

19. Cover continue to cook to absorb excess liquid and both the rice and lentils are well cooked in 20 minutes.

20. Let it rest undisturbed and covered for 5 minutes.

21. Make the pasta accordingly to the manufacturers package Directions.

22. Drain any excess water.

23. Cover the chickpeas and warm in the microwave shortly.

24. Next, fluff the rice and lentils with a fork.

25. Shift to a serving platter.

26. Then, Top with the elbow pasta and tomato sauce, chickpeas also crispy onions for purposes of garnishing.

27. Serve and enjoy.

Mediterranean pan seared sea bass recipe with a garlic bell pepper medley

Ingredients

- ½ tablespoon of garlic powder
- 4 pieces of Sea Bass fillet, no skin
- 1 teaspoon of Aleppo pepper
- 3 cups of cooked rice
- Salt
- Extra virgin olive oil
- 1 Green Bell Pepper, cored and chopped
- 1 Red Bell Pepper, cored and chopped
- ½ lemon, juice off
- 1 teaspoon of ground cumin
- 3 Shallots, chopped
- ½ teaspoon of black pepper
- 4 garlic cloves, minced
- ½ cup of pitted Kalamata olives, halved
- ½ tablespoon of ground coriander

Directions

1. Take the fish out of the fridge about 20 minutes before cooking. Sprinkle with salt on both sides and set aside.
2. In a small bowl, combine the spices to make the spice mixture. Also set aside for later.
3. In a medium-sized skillet, heat 2 tablespoon of olive oil over medium-high heat until shimmering but with no smoke.
4. Add the bell peppers together with the shallots and garlic.
5. Season with salt and spice mixture you prepared earlier.
6. Let cook for 5 minutes as you stir regularly until the peppers have softened.
7. Lower the heat stir in the chopped olives.
8. Leave on low heat as fish gets ready.
9. Pat fish dry and season with the remaining spice mixture.
10. In a large skillet, heat ¼ cup of extra virgin olive oil over medium-high until shimmering but with no smoke.
11. Add the fish pieces.
12. Push to the middle for 30 seconds.
13. Let cook on one side, undisturbed, until nicely browned not longer than 6 minutes.
14. Turn the fish over and cook on other side for the same until nicely browned as well.
15. Remove fish from source of heat.
16. Drizzle with lemon juice.

17. Serve hot and enjoy with the bell pepper medley spooned on top as well as cooked couscous.

Persian baked omelet

Ingredients

- ¼ teaspoon of ground black pepper
- 2 cups of flat-leaf parsley, leaves
- ½ cup of walnuts, toasted and chopped
- 2 cups of cilantro, leaves and tender stems
- 1 cup of roughly chopped fresh dill
- ½ teaspoon of ground cumin
- ⅓ cup of dried cranberries, coarsely chopped
- 5 tablespoons of Greek extra virgin olive oil
- 6 scallions, trimmed and coarsely chopped
- 1 ½ teaspoons of baking powder
- 1 teaspoon of kosher salt
- ¾ teaspoon of ground green cardamom
- 6 large eggs
- ¾ teaspoon of ground cinnamon

Directions

1. Position an oven rack in the upper-middle position and heat oven to 375 °F.
2. Trace the bottom of a square pan, then cut inside the lines to create a piece to fit in the bottom of the pan.

3. Coat the bottom and sides of the pan with 2 tablespoons of extra virgin olive oil, turning the parchment to coat on both sides.

4. In a food processor, combine the parsley together with the cilantro, dill, scallions, and remaining 3 tablespoons of extra virgin olive oil.

5. Process until finely ground and keep aside for later.

6. In a large bowl, whisk the baking powder together with the salt, cardamom, cinnamon, cumin and pepper.

7. Add 2 eggs and whisk until blended.

8. Add the remaining eggs and whisk until just combined.

9. Fold in the herb-scallion mixture and the walnuts together with the cranberries.

10. Pour into the prepared pan and smooth the top.

11. Let bake at 375°F until the center of the egg is firm in 25 minutes.

12. Let the kuku cool in the pan undisturbed for 10 minutes.

13. Run a thin knife around the edges to loosen the kuku.

14. Then, invert onto a plate and remove the parchment from bottom.

15. Re-invert on another serving plate so the top of the kuku is facing up.

16. Slice into wedges and serve warm.

17. You can serve with a dollop of yogurt.

18. Enjoy.

Lentil Bolognese sauce

If you are looking for a nutrient packed and rich flavor dish, then do not look further. The lentil Bolognese sauce is deliciously flavored with onions, herbs and celery which can be serves with spaghetti.

Ingredients

- 1 cup Water
- 1 Medium Onion, minced
- 1 can Crushed Tomatoes
- 1 Large Carrot, finely diced
- 4 Garlic Cloves, minced
- 2 tablespoons Olive Oil
- 1.5 cup Cooked Lentils
- ½ teaspoon Salt
- 2 teaspoons Dried Basil
- 1 Large Celery, finely diced
- 1/8 teaspoon Black Pepper

Directions

1. In a medium pot, heat the oil.

2. Add minced diced celery, onion, and diced carrot.

3. Sauté on medium-high temperature for 10 minutes keep stirring frequently.

4. Add the minced garlic then stir for 1 minute.

5. Pour 1 cup of water together with the remaining ingredients mainly cooked lentils, salt, crushed tomatoes, pepper and dried basil. Stir properly.

6. Boil let simmer over reduced temperature till when the carrots and celery are completely cooked in 25 minutes.

7. Serve and enjoy.

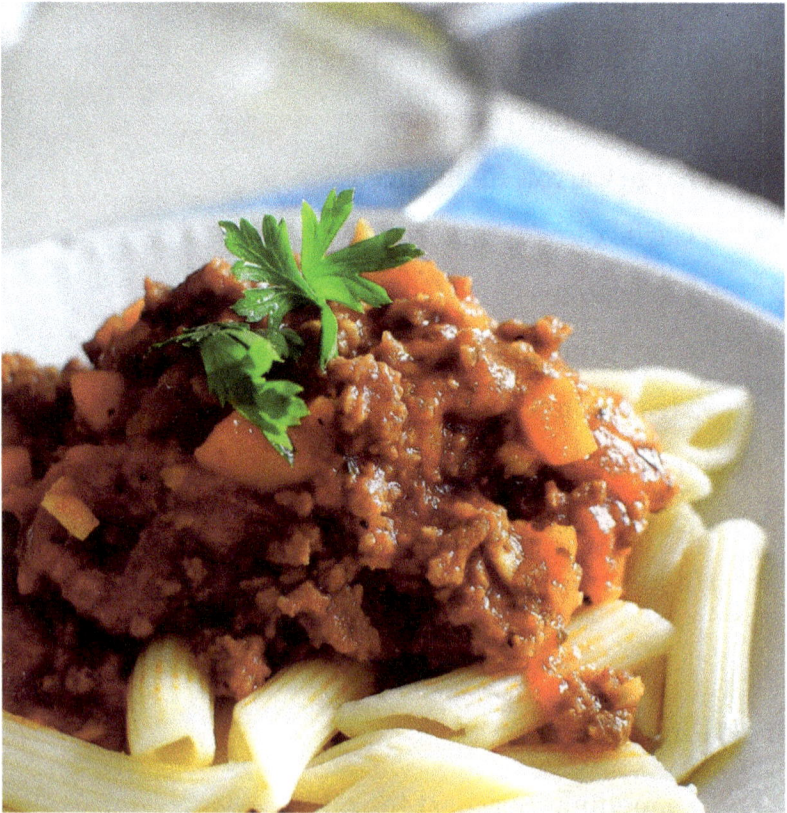

Homemade vegetable lasagna

Prepared with massive variety of vegetables served with white sauce, this recipe is healthy enough for anyone who loves Mediterranean Sea diet.

Ingredients

- 10 Lasagna Sheets
- 1 ounce of Butter
- 2 Large Celery Stalks, finely diced
- ½ cups Half and Half
- 1 tablespoon Dried Oregano
- Cheese of your choice
- 2 Zucchinis, diced (6 cups)
- 3 tablespoons Double Concentrated Tomato Puree
- 1 can Plum Tomatoes
- 1 teaspoon Salt
- 1 tablespoon Dried Basil
- 1/3 cup of All-Purpose Flour
- 2 Medium Onions minced
- 3 Bell Peppers diced
- Pinch of Salt
- 1.5 cups Milk

- Pinch of Black Pepper
- ¼ teaspoon Black Pepper

Directions

1. In a large pot, heat oil then, introduce in the onions, chopped peppers, celery and zucchini.
2. Sauté for 10 minutes as you stir frequently.
3. Preheat the oven to 200° as you soak the lasagna sheets.
4. Melting butter in a small sauce pan for preparing white sauce.
5. Stir in flour and pour in milk half by half as you regularly stir.
6. Bring to a boil.
7. Reduce the heat and simmer until the sauce becomes thick enough.
8. Put off the heat and set aside.
9. Add plum tomatoes, tomato puree, pepper, salt, basil and oregano to the pot when the vegetables are ready.
10. When the veggies are ready, mix to combined.
11. Cook for more 5 minutes and turn off heat when ready
12. Get an oven proof dish and cover the bottom with lasagna sheets.
13. Spread a good layer of white sauce over and top with 1/3 of the vegetable mixture.
14. Repeat the process for 2 more times.

15. Cover the last layer of veggies with a layer of lasagna sheets and top with cheese.
16. Bake in a preheated oven for 30 minutes until the sheets and veggies are cooked and cheese turn golden brown.
17. Remove the lasagna from the oven let settle for 10 – 15 minutes
18. Serve and enjoy

Broccoli curry

This recipe is ideal for the busiest families with limited time as it only gets ready in 25 minutes. Above and beyond, anyone can make this recipe easily.

Ingredients

- A drizzle of lemon juice
- 1 medium onion, finely minced
- 1/8 teaspoon black pepper
- 1 teaspoon salt
- 1 teaspoon ground ginger
- 1.5 cups of vegetable broth
- 1 can of coconut milk
- 1 tablespoon olive oil
- 4 garlic cloves
- 2 cups of cooked lentils
- 2 tablespoons mild curry powder
- 6 cups of raw broccoli florets

Directions

1. In a large pot, heat oil.

2. Add minced onion then sauté for 2 minutes.

3. Add minced garlic and stir well to release the aroma

4. Add curry powder together with ginger, stir briefly.

5. Add broccoli florets, broth, lentils, coconut milk, and salt and pepper and stir well to combine.

6. Bring to a boil.

7. Reduce the heat allow to simmer for 10 – 15 minutes.

8. Add a drizzle of lemon juice

9. Serve and enjoy with rice.

10. 1055. Homemade tuna pizza

11. A handful pantry is all you need to make this deliciously sweet tuna pizza. The dough and sauce can be made easily from scratch.

12. Ingredients

13. Fresh basil leaves

14. 1 pound pizza dough

15. ½ cup sweetcorn

16. 1 cup shredded cheese

17. 3 tablespoons pizza sauce

18. 5 ounces canned tuna, drained

19. Directions

20. Start by rolling out the pizza dough.

21. Move the dough onto a baking sheet lined with baking parchment paper when it is ready.

22. Top it with the sauce (half), tuna, shredded cheese, and sweetcorn.

23. Repeat this process for all the pizza.

24. Bake in the oven over 200° for 10 minutes or more accordingly.

25. Serve warm and enjoy.

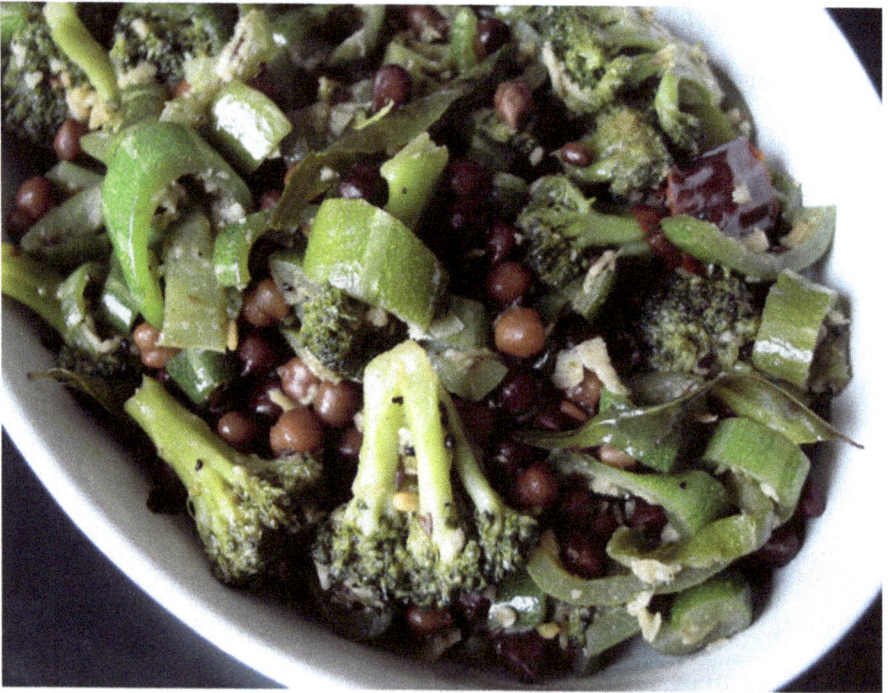

Cauliflower chicken curry

Do not be surprised to realize the truth that this is an onion free recipe but it has other flavorful ingredients like milk. Still, this is a perfect dinner for a weeknight.

Ingredients

- 1/8 teaspoon of black pepper
- 1 tablespoon of olive oil
- 3 tablespoons of mild curry powder
- 1 can coconut milk
- 1 pound of cauliflower florets
- 1 teaspoon of ground ginger
- 1.5 cup of low sodium vegetable broth
- 1 teaspoon of salt
- 1 can of tomato passata
- 4 garlic cloves
- 1.5 cup of cooked chickpeas

Directions

1. Ultimately, start by heating the oil in a large pot.
2. Add crushed garlic and sauté until aromatic for 1 minute.

3. Add curry powder together with the ginger stir for up to 30 seconds to combine.

4. Add the broth, coconut milk, passata, cooked chickpeas, cauliflower florets, salt and pepper stir to combine then cover well.

5. Reduce the heat let simmer for 15 minutes

6. Uncover let simmer for more 10 minutes until tender.

7. You can cook longer that 10 minutes according to how you want it.

8. Remove from the heat source, let cool.

9. Serve and enjoy.

Tuna burrito

The tuna burrito is a perfect meal for lunch, dinner and also as a snack.

Ingredients

- shredded cheese
- ½ English cucumber
- 8 ounces canned tuna
- ½ cup celery
- ½ cup mayonnaise
- 1.5 cups cooked rice
- ⅓ cup yellow onion minced
- salt
- black pepper
- ½ cup canned sweetcorn
- 4 flour tortillas

Directions

1. Combine together sweetcorn, drained tuna, chopped celery, mayonnaise, rice, minced onion, salt and pepper in a mixing bowl mix properly.

2. Taste and season accordingly.
3. Place 10 slices of cucumber in the center of tortilla rows.
4. Cover well with a quarter of the tuna filling.
5. Sprinkle with cheese (though optional)
6. Roll into burrito
7. Wrap the ends in aluminum foil and cut in half
8. Serve and enjoy.

Creamy tuna pasta bake

In about 35 minutes this tuna pasta will be ready waiting for your bite for a weeknight dinner. This casserole can feed a family of up to six people without having to struggle to make it.

Ingredients

- ¾ cup of half and half
- 1.5 cup of broccoli florets (75g)
- ½ cup of sour cream
- salt
- ½ teaspoon of celery salt
- 10 ounces of short pasta (300g)
- ¼ teaspoon of ground black pepper
- 7 ounces canned of tuna, drained (200g)
- 1.5 tablespoon of herbs de Provence
- 5 ounces of canned sweet corn, drained
- 7 ounces of cheese, shredded or sliced (200g)

Directions

1. Firstly, cook pasta according to package Directions.
2. When it is about to cool, add broccoli florets.

3. Cook until both the pasta and broccoli are ready.

4. Drain excess water.

5. Preheat the oven to 200° as the pasta cooks.

6. Mix together about an ounce of shredded cheese with half and half as well as sour cream.

7. Keep aside.

8. Put the pasta and broccoli back into the same pot

9. Add celery, salt, herbs de Provence, sweetcorn, black pepper, tuna and the sour cream mixture blend well to combined.

10. Transfer to a casserole dish adequate enough to accommodate the mixture.

11. Cover with cheese

12. Bake in a preheated oven for 20 minutes or more accordingly.

13. Serve and enjoy.

Pressure cranberry chicken

Ingredients

- 2 tablespoons of all-purpose flour
- 1 small onion, minced
- black pepper
- 2 ounces of pancetta
- 1 cup of frozen cranberries
- 4 chicken thighs, skinless, bone-in
- 1.5 teaspoon salt
- ⅔ cup of vegetable broth
- ½ cup of cranberry sauce
- ½ teaspoon of paprika
- 2 tablespoons of olive oil
- 3 orange slices, optional

Directions

1. Turn on Pressure pot.
2. Instruct accordingly, then pour olive oil and Sauté as you peel and cut the onion.
3. Add it to the pot and Sauté for 2 minutes until translucent.
4. Add bacon or the pancetta pieces let fry for 2 minutes.

5. On the other hand, keep seasoning the thighs with salt, paprika, and black pepper.
6. Create space in the pot
7. Add the chicken cook for 2 minutes on every side.
8. Disable the Sauté function
9. Deglaze the pot with broth
10. Introduce the cranberry sauce while stirring until well combined.
11. Add half of the cranberries together 2 – 3 orange slices.
12. Tightly close the lid under lock in a firm position.
13. Release the valve to seal the content inside for 6 minute as timed on the timer.
14. After the time has run out, let simmer for 4 – 5 minutes. Then release the pressure.
15. Reduce the lid after the pin drops
16. Turn back on the Sauté function.
17. Add cranberries and make sure the sauce thickens with flour measured in 2 tablespoons blended with water.
18. cook for 1 - 2 minutes then turn off the pot.
19. Serve and enjoy with rice.

Pressure pot pasta with mushroom and spinach

The Pressure pot pasta is another dish for busy families as it does not consume much time to get ready for a bite. It is best prepared with a pressure cooker for the pasta.

Ingredients

- 1 tablespoon of dried oregano
- A pinch of salt
- 1 small onion
- 3 garlic cloves, minced
- 1 tablespoon of Worcestershire sauce
- 2½ cups of vegetable broth
- ½ cup of sweet corn
- 1/3 cup of parmesan cheese
- ½ cup of pitted green olives
- A pinch of black pepper
- 6 ounces of button mushrooms
- ½ cup of half and half (120 ml)
- 1 tablespoon of oil
- 6 ounces of short-shaped pasta
- 3 handfuls of fresh spinach

Directions

1. Pour oil into the stainless-steel insert.
2. Turn on the Sauté function.
3. Add minced onion and quartered mushrooms.
4. Sauté for about 3 minutes as you keep stirring occasionally.
5. Add minced garlic and stir for only 1 minute to prevent burning and ensure proper release of aroma.
6. Add olives, Worcestershire sauce, stock, oregano, pasta, black pepper and salt do not forget to mix properly.
7. With a spatula, push down the pasta.
8. Close with a lid and lock it firmly in position.
9. Set timer according to pasta cooking Directions on the package.
10. Divide this time by two and subtract 2 minutes for accurate cooking time estimation.
11. Release the pressure manually if the cooking cycle is complete.
12. Remove the lid and Sauté again.
13. Pour in half and half and cook until the sauce thickens somehow.
14. Finally, stir in sweet corn together with the spinach and Parmesan cheese.
15. Remove from the pot.
16. Serve and enjoy.

Zucchini lasagna

The zucchini lasagna is baked to perfection after it is layered on every side with meaty and mozzarella. It might take up to 50 minutes to 1 hour to get ready so you have to be put as your deal with your taste buds awakened by the aromatic flavors in the recipe.

Ingredient

- 2 medium zucchini, sliced
- ¼ teaspoon of ground black pepper
- 1 small onion, minced
- Mozzarella slices
- 2 bay leaves
- 14 ounce of ground beef
- ½ teaspoon of salt
- 2 teaspoon of dried oregano
- 1 can crushed tomatoes
- ½ teaspoon of ground cinnamon
- 1 tablespoon of extra virgin olive oil
- 1 teaspoon of garlic powder
- 4 ounces tomato puree (90g)

Directions

1. Expressly, begin by trimming off the ends of each zucchini
2. Then cut the zucchini in half.
3. Place the cut side onto a chopping board and cut each half into thin slices.
4. Place all the cut zucchini onto a tray and sprinkle salt over.
5. Keep all of them aside.
6. Preheat the oven ready to 200°.
7. In a heavy skillet, heat oil, later when shimmered without smoke, add minced onion in.
8. Sauté for 3 minutes or so
9. Add ½ tsp of salt, garlic powder, ground beef, cinnamon, black pepper, oregano and bay leaves.
10. Break the ground meat then season when everything is properly mixed making sure the seasoning is evenly distributed.
11. Cook for 5 minutes.
12. Stir in crushed tomatoes together with the tomato puree
13. Cook until the sauce thickens with minimal liquid.
14. Pat dry zucchini slices.
15. Assemble the lasagna
16. Cover the bottom of an oven-proof dish with the zucchini slices.

17. Top them with a thin layer of meat sauce and mozzarella cheese.
18. Repeat this process till you have all the zucchini slices are used up together the meat sauce.
19. You should have 3 layers of zucchini, 2 layers of cheese and 3 layers of meat sauce.
20. Keep the leftover cheese for later.
21. Bake in the preheated oven for 15 minutes.
22. Remove from the oven, top with mozzarella cheese and return to the oven for more 10 minutes cooking
23. Allow it to settle for 15 minutes when ready.
24. Serve and enjoy.

Pressure pot zucchini mushroom risotto

This dish is particularly convenient and a perfect match with summer rice. Besides, the zucchini mushroom risotto does not involve standing the whole day waiting for it to get ready. It is a quick dish in about 15 minutes max.

Ingredients

- 1 small onion chopped
- Unsalted butter
- 2 tablespoons of Worcestershire sauce
- 1 cup of arborio rice
- 4 ounces of button mushrooms
- 2 teaspoons of dried oregano
- 3 garlic cloves, minced
- 1.5 cup of vegetable broth
- Fresh chives chopped (optional)
- 3 tablespoons of extra virgin olive oil
- Black pepper
- ¼ cup of red wine
- 2 cups of zucchini chunks (220 grams)
- 1 teaspoon salt

- Parmesan cheese

Directions

1. Prep all the ingredients.
2. Turn on the Pressure pot and select the option to Sauté.
3. Pour the oil inside the stainless steel pot
4. And the chopped onion.
5. Sauté until translucent.
6. Add mushrooms and garlic while stirring constantly for 1 minute.
7. Add red wine and mix blend.
8. Allow to cook for 2 – 3 minutes to evaporate the alcohol.
9. Add salt, Worcestershire sauce, pepper, rice, zucchini, oregano and vegetable broth and mix thoroughly then cover tightly.
10. Seal with the steam valve let cook at a high temperature for 3 minutes.
11. When the time is up, switch off, release the pressure.
12. Finally, stir in Parmesan, butter, and fresh chives
13. Serve and enjoy.

Mediterranean grilled vegetables

This recipe follows the heart of true Mediterranean Sea diet because of plenty of veggies seasoned and grilled to expected perfection. More so, it can be adjusted according to how one likes to enjoy it.

Ingredients

- 2 tablespoons of Oregano
- 1 Green Bell Pepper
- 1 tsp Salt
- 4 oz. Button Mushrooms
- 2 tablespoons of Olive Oil
- 1 Large Red Onion
- 1 Yellow Bell Pepper
- 1 cup Cherry Tomatoes
- 1 Zucchini
- Black Pepper

Directions

1. Wash and rinse all the vegetables and cut them into chunks except the button mushrooms which must be cut

in half, onion into quarters make sure to separate the layers.

2. Place all the vegetables onto a baking tray apart from cherry tomatoes.

3. Season with pepper, salt, oregano and olive oil mix to combine and mix and check to see everything is coated

4. Grill for 10 minutes as you stir occasionally.

5. Add the cherry tomatoes to grill for more 10 minutes.

6. Serve and enjoy.

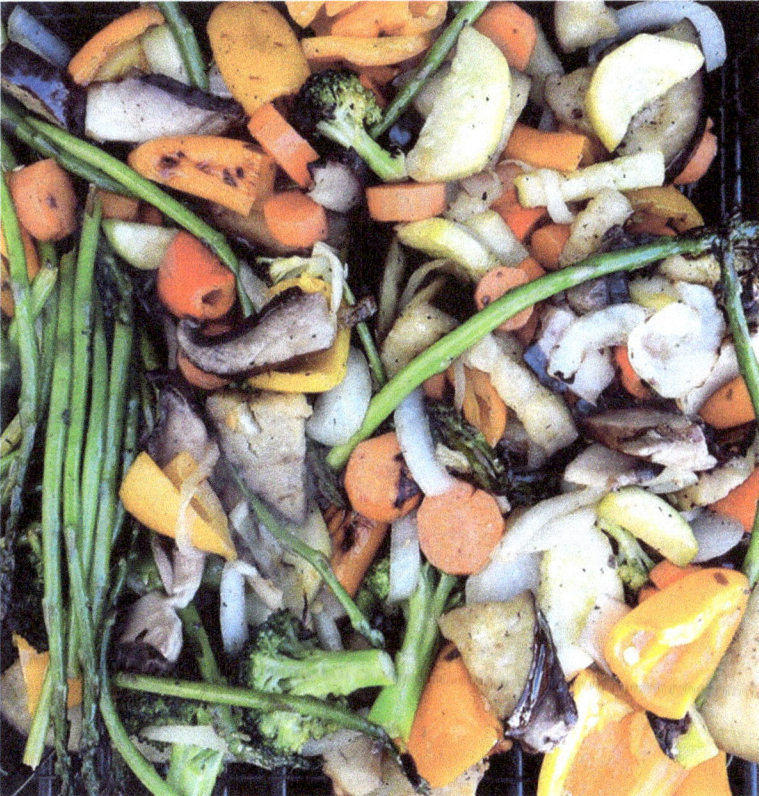

Ash roasted potatoes

No stress of move to all stores to seek for several ingredients, this recipe only has one ingredient largely the potato. The outcome is a soft smoky potato on the inside. Nevertheless, one can decide to enjoy with their favorite Mediterranean Sea diet sauce.

Ingredients

- Sour Cream
- 4 Medium Potatoes
- Black Pepper
- Salt
- Butter

Directions

1. Definitely, start by thoroughly washing the potatoes
2. Wrap every potato well in a sheet of aluminum foil.
3. Bury the potatoes in the ashes and let them cook for 60 - 89 minutes.
4. Unwrap to see if they are full ready.
5. Ensure the potatoes are somewhat black on the outside.
6. Remove and enjoy when warm.

Easy campfire potatoes

Why should you be bored in your camp? Light up some fire and roast potatoes with onions, parmesan and rosemary. Check out the recipe.

Ingredients

- 4 tablespoon of Butter
- 1 Onion
- 2 lbs. Potatoes
- 1 teaspoon of Paprika
- 1.5 teaspoon of Salt
- ¼ teaspoon of Black Pepper
- 2 Fresh Rosemary Sprigs

Directions

1. Wash the potatoes thoroughly in a running water after, cut into chunks.
2. Move into a large bowl.
3. Add the seasoning and toss the potatoes until potatoes are well coated.
4. Peel and cut the onion in half, further cut the halves into slices.

5. Separate the slices and add them to the bowl altogether with rosemary mix well.
6. Divide the potatoes in 4 sheets of aluminum foil.
7. Top each with a tablespoon of butter and wrap in the foil.
8. Cook in the ashes or just on a grill depending on what is convenient for you for 30 – 40 minutes.
9. Open the packets and sprinkle with Parmesan.
10. Serve when still warm and enjoy.

Buffalo chicken tacos

Like many other recipes, this buffalo is highly customizable to individual preference. So, no need to worry about rigidity.

Ingredients

- Buffalo sauce
- ¼ cup of hot sauce
- Grated cheese
- 3 tablespoon of cilantro, chopped
- 1 cup of Greek yogurt
- 1 tablespoon of honey
- 2 tablespoon of honey
- 2 limes, juice only
- 12 small tortillas
- ½ stick unsalted butter
- 2 cups of shredded rotisserie chicken
- 2 ripe medium avocados
- Fresh cilantro
- ½ head iceberg lettuce, shredded
- 2 - 3 spring onions
- Lime wedges

Directions

1. Boil the sauce in a small sauce pan.

2. Reduce the heat to allow it to simmer for 1 minute as you keep stirring constantly.

3. Remove from the heat and stir in honey and butter until melted.

4. In a mixing bowl, combine the sauce together shredded chicken.

5. In a small bowl, mix all the ingredients until well combined to make the cilantro sauce.

6. Place the tortillas on a tray and top all of them with shredded buffalo chicken, lettuce, spring onions, avocado slices, some cilantro leaves and sprinkle with cheese.

7. Drizzle each taco with the cilantro sauce.

8. Serve immediately and enjoy.

Easy shepherd's pie

The ease with which this dish is made in approximately 1 hour makes it a perfect choice for a family. Hearty vegetables topped with massive meat pie and smashed makes it a powerful energy sauce.

Ingredients

- 1.5 teaspoon of salt
- ¾ stick of unsalted butter (80g)
- 5 tablespoon of tomato puree
- 1 cup of frozen peas
- 2 tablespoon of oil see note 3
- 1 medium onion diced
- Black pepper
- 2.2 pounds of potatoes
- Salt
- Black pepper
- 2 cups of water (500ml)
- 1 lb. ground beef (450g)
- 5 tablespoon of Worcestershire sauce
- 2 cups of chicken stock
- ½ cup milk (120ml)

- 2 medium carrots diced
- 2 teaspoons of dried thyme

Directions

1. Put the diced potatoes into a pot.
2. Add salt and cover with water.
3. Boil with the lid covered well.
4. Lower the heat to allow it to simmer while covered till soft.
5. Drain the water when ready
6. Add butter and milk and mash until smooth keep for later.
7. In a large skillet, heat the oil until shimmering without smoke.
8. Sauté carrots and onion for 5 minutes after which add ground beef.
9. Break up the meat and cook for 5 minutes, keep stirring occasionally.
10. Add Worcestershire sauce, tomato puree, thyme, chicken stock, pinch of salt and pepper to the content let mix.
11. Lower the heat and continue to cook for 20 minutes.
12. Stir in the peas, then cover with potato mash when ready when done.
13. Bake in already heated oven 200° for 30 minutes.
14. Serve while warm and enjoy.

Sweet potato gnocchi

This potato is perfectly served with parmesan and green pesto. In only 12 minutes it is not difficult to hold your hunger longer for its bite.

Ingredients

- 1 cup of mashed sweet potato
- 1 cup of all-purpose flour
- Pinch of Salt
- Extra for water
- 1 small of Egg
- Oil for frying, optional
- 2 tablespoons of Green Pesto
- Parmesan

Instruction

1. Boil salted water in a large pot.
2. As the salted water boils, combine together cold mashed sweet potato, flour and salt on a clean work surface.
3. Make a well like deepening in the middle to pour the beaten egg.
4. Using a fork mix everything together.

5. Then knead to form dough in utmost 2 minutes.

6. Cut the dough into 8 pieces.

7. Dust your work and top with flour.

8. Roll pieces into a sausage thinner than a cigar.

9. Cut them into small pieces.

10. Cook in a large pot with the already salted boiling water for 2 minutes until when they start floating on top.

11. Serve them either boiled or pan-roasted with a sauce of your liking

12. Enjoy.

Corned beef mashed potatoes

This Mediterranean Sea diet is a perfect side dish options with packed flavors especially dill pickles, jalapenos, milk among others.

Ingredients

- ¼ cup of dill pickles
- 1¼ lbs. of potatoes (600g)
- 2 teaspoon of butter (30g)
- Fresh parsley
- 1 teaspoon of salt
- ½ cup of milk
- 7 ounces canned corned beef
- ¼ cup of jalapenos , drained, sliced

Directions

1. Wash, peel and cut the potatoes into small pieces.
2. Move the cut potatoes into a pot and pour water over just cover them all.
3. Add salt.
4. Cover the pot with a lid and bring to a boil.

5. Lower the temperature once boiling starts to let simmer until they are all cooked through.
6. Drain any excess water.
7. Mash the potatoes using a potato masher.
8. Add milk and butter blend well until well combined and smooth.
9. Add and mix in the corned beef.
10. Cut the jalapenos, dill pickles, and parsley.
11. Stir them together into the mash and garnish with fresh parsley.
12. Serve warm and enjoy.

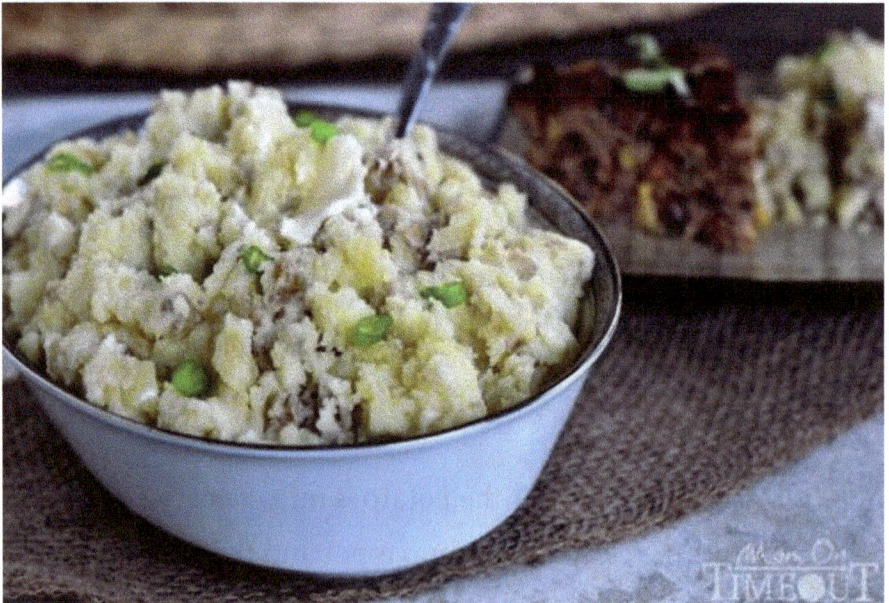

Lentil curry recipe

Lentil curry is perfectly prepared as potato lentil curry in an Pressure pot. Sweet potatoes will always jubilate when encountered with potatoes and lentil prepared following this recipe.

Ingredients

- 13 ounces of coconut milk
- 3 teaspoons of Thai curry paste
- 1 large onion, chopped
- 3 tablespoons of olive oil
- 1 teaspoons of cumin powder
- 1 cup of uncooked lentils
- 1 teaspoons of ginger
- 13 ounces of tomato passatta
- 1 teaspoons of turmeric powder
- Avocado
- 1 garlic clove
- 1 teaspoons of salt
- Parsley
- 1 large sweet potato
- 2 tablespoons of concentrated tomato puree

- Chili

Directions

1. Start by turning on the Sauté functionality on Pressure pot.
2. Add in the olive oil together with the chopped onion.
3. Then Sauté until the onion turns translucent in 4 minutes.
4. Add the pressed garlic and stir for 1 minute.
5. Switch off the Sauté functionality.
6. Add the rest of the ingredients and one and half cup of water.
7. Lock the lid firmly.
8. Then turn on the steam valve to enable sealing.
9. Set time to 4 minutes.
10. Wait for extra 10 minutes when the time has run up before you can release the pressure.
11. Serve when still warm with quinoa, rice, naan bread.
12. You can also add avocado, parsley and chili as desired.

Vietnamese sandwich banh mi

Forget the Vietnamese name, this is a healthy Mediterranean Sea diet packed and stuffed with huge variety of veggies, cold cuts and cilantro. Make it home following the step by step procedures below.

Ingredients

- 1 daikon (60 grams)
- 1 carrot
- Fresh cilantro
- 1 small chili pepper or jalapeno to taste
- 2-3 tablespoons white wine vinegar
- 2 French baguette rolls
- 2 tablespoons pate
- 1 cucumber
- 2 teaspoons Thai red curry paste
- 4 tablespoons mayonnaise
- 8 slices cold cuts

Directions

1. The carrots and daikon must be peeled and washed.

2. Cut them carefully into matchsticks and place into a bowl.

3. Add the vinegar over and set aside for later.

4. Mix mayonnaise with red curry paste.

5. Cut open the baguettes.

6. Spread one side with pate and the other side with the mayonnaise mixture.

7. Divide all the fillings equally in between the two baguettes.

8. Drain out excess vinegar.

9. Add the pickled vegetables.

10. Serve and enjoy.

Pressure pot stuffed tomatoes

Stuffed tomatoes are stuffed with meat and rice topped with breadcrumbs and cheese to make a complete meal for lunch of dinner and or heavy breakfast option in lesser time of 17 minutes.

Ingredients

- 8 tomatoes on vine
- 7 ounces of ground beef
- 1 tablespoon of sunflower oil
- ½ teaspoon of salt
- Pinch of black pepper
- 3 teaspoons of dried oregano
- ½ teaspoon of garlic powder
- 1¼ cup of cooked rice
- 3 ounces of feta cheese
- ¼ cup of fresh parsley, chopped
- 1 ounce of cheddar cheese, grated
- 3 tablespoons of breadcrumbs

Directions

1. Slice off the top of every tomato and set aside for later.
2. Using a teaspoon, scoop out the seeds and pulp and put them into a food processor.
3. After blending, transfer into the inner pot of the Pressure pot.
4. In a skillet, cook the ground beef with small oil, black pepper, salt, and garlic powder and season well for even distribution while stirring.
5. When the beef is cooked, transfer to the mixing bowl.
6. Add crumbled Feta cheese, cooked rice, and chopped parsley.
7. Mix together until well combined, taste and season accordingly.
8. In a small bowl, mix the breadcrumbs with grated cheddar also keep aside.
9. Get the tomatoes and stuff each of them with the ground beef mixture, top them with the breadcrumb put in the Pressure pot.
10. Place the tops back on the tomatoes.
11. Lock the lid in a stable and firm position.
12. Set time to 2 minutes run the cooker.
13. Release the pressure immediately when the time is up.
14. Serve and enjoy.

Pressure pot stuffed with sweet potatoes

Ingredients

- 1 lemon
- 2 medium sweet potatoes
- 3 ounces of feta cheese (90 grams)
- 2 spring onions
- Olive oil
- Cup of cooked couscous (140 grams)
- Salt and pepper to taste
- 1 cup of cooked chickpeas
- 1 teaspoon of paprika
- 1 avocado

Directions

1. Wash the sweet potatoes thoroughly under running water.
2. Pierce them with a knife.
3. Place 1½ cup of water into the of the electric pressure cooker.
4. Insert the steam rack for putting sweet potatoes.
5. Lock the lid in its position firmly.

6. Turn the steam release valve to seal.

7. Adjust timer to 17 minutes over pressure.

8. As the timer runs up, pan-roast the drained chickpeas with some olive oil.

9. Add salt and pepper and season, stir to evenly coat the chickpeas. When you see the chickpeas turn to brown, add paprika and stir again.

10. Turn off the heat and cut the spring onions.

11. Peel and cut the avocado in half and slice.

12. When the sweet potatoes are ready, hold on until the steam is released by itself in 4 – 5 minutes.

13. Turn off the pressure cooker and open the lid.

14. Let the potatoes cool down briefly, cut in half lengthwise.

15. Mash the inside with a fork mainly to create space for the toppings.

16. Add the toppings

17. Serve and enjoy with lemon wedges and crumbled Feta.

Cabbage and sausage foil packets

The recipe takes preparation of cabbage to the next level. They are cooked in packets in the oven which makes it conducive for outdoor cooking especially grilling in 55 minutes.

Ingredients

- 1 teaspoon of salt
- ¼ teaspoon of black pepper
- 11 ounces of white cabbage
- 10 baby potatoes
- 1½ teaspoon of caraway seeds , crushed
- 1 large onion
- 3 ounces of Italian sausage
- a handful of fresh parsley
- 3 tablespoons of extra virgin olive oil

Directions

1. Chop the cabbage in a rough manner.
2. Cut the potatoes and sausages into chunks.
3. Cut the onion into quarters and separate the layers.
4. Move everything into a large bowl

5. Add chopped parsley and season with pepper, salt, caraway seeds.

6. Drizzle with olive oil and carefully toss the salad until all the ingredients are well coated.

7. Move the mixture to 4 large sheets of foil.

8. Wrap each pocket well without holes.

9. Bake in an oven at 200° for 30 – 35 minutes

10. Serve and enjoy.

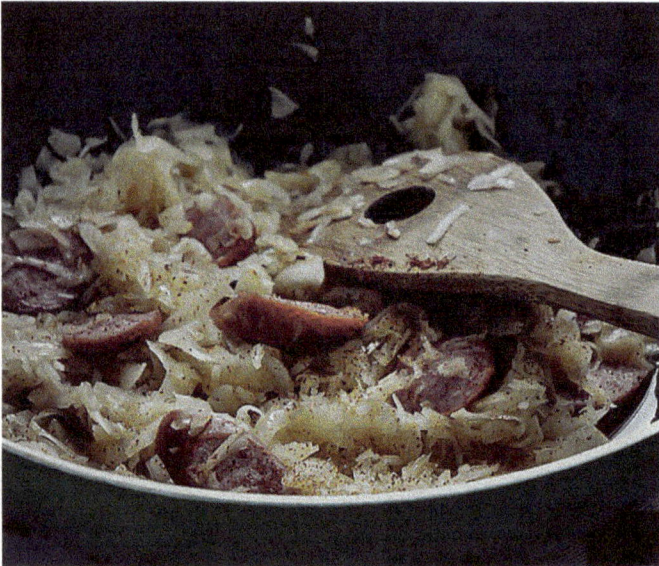

Skillet chicken fajitas

This healthy chicken recipe is stuffed with many flavors and gets ready in 15 minutes, therefore you need not to worry about waiting for your meal the whole day. the chicken is juicy seasoned with veggies crunchy enough to shoot up your taste buds.

Ingredients

- Fajita seasoning
- Salt and pepper
- 8 flour tortillas
  o ounces of chicken breasts
- 4 teaspoon of olive oil
- 3 bell peppers
- A handful of cilantro
- 2.5 tablespoon of ketchup
- 2 garlic cloves
- 5 tablespoons of Greek yogurt
- 1 medium onion
- 2 large avocados

Directions

1. Cut the chicken breast into thin strips immediately season with fajita then keep aside for later.

2. Peel and cut the onion into quarters do not forget to separate the layers

3. Cut the peppers into thin strips.

4. Heat the olive oil in a large skillet until shimmering without smoke, add the onion and peppers.

5. Season with small salt and pepper as you stir fry on high temperature for 3 minutes.

6. Tossing occasionally.

7. Move into a bowl.

8. Add oil to the skillet followed with the seasoned chicken strips

9. Stir fry until they have cooked through.

10. Place the veggies back into the pan, toss until warm.

11. Mix the ketchup together with the Greek yogurt and minced garlic.

12. Serve with avocados, tortillas, and cilantro.

13. Enjoy.

Spinach and asparagus frittata

This largely a light and fluffy recipe with spinach and asparagus for veggie lovers. It is fully packed with vegetables making a healthy meal for your family.

Ingredients

- ½ teaspoon of salt
- 3 tablespoons of olive oil
- A pinch of black pepper
- 1 small onion, diced
- 2 teaspoons of dried thyme
- 3 ounces of cheddar cheese
- 7 ounce of fresh asparagus stalks
- 5 medium eggs
- 7 ounce of fresh spinach
- ½ cup of milk
- 3 garlic cloves

Directions

1. Heat oil and add diced onion in an oven-proof skillet.
2. Sauté for 1 minute then add the spinach.

3. Sauté until when the spinach has significantly reduced its volume.
4. Preheat your oven to 200°.
5. As the oven is heating, wash the asparagus and trim off the hard ends.
6. Cut the rest of the stalks into 1-inch-long pieces.
7. Peel and mince the garlic.
8. Add both the garlic and asparagus to the spinach, sauté for 1 – 2 minutes.
9. In a medium sized bowl, beat the eggs.
10. Add pepper, thyme, salt, and milk blend well.
11. Pour it gently over the veggies and cook briefly.
12. Move the skillet into the oven typically when the eggs around the edges start to set,
13. Bake for 15 minutes
14. Top with grated cheese
15. Serve warm and enjoy for lunch or any meal time.

Spinach and cheddar quiche

Enjoy this absolutely meat free pie recipe possible to serve as an appetizer or main dish as well. It is fully stuffed with veggies, cream mixture, and an egg topped with cheese achieve the sweetness that you are seeking for in 50 minutes.

Ingredients

- 2 eggs
- 1½ cup of all-purpose flour
- 1 leek
- ½ stick of unsalted butter
- 1 small egg
- ¼ teaspoon of black pepper
- 3 tablespoons of cold water
- ¾ cup of milk
- 2 teaspoons of vegetable oil
- A pinch of salt
- 2 cups pf frozen spinach
- ½ teaspoon of salt
- ½ cup of half and half
- 1 small red onion
- 2 ounces of grated cheese

Directions

1. Start with the crust, therefore, Place flour, chilled diced butter, and salt in a food processor.
2. Process until crumb-like texture.
3. Add the egg and cold water continue to process until the dough pulls together.
4. Remove out and wrap in a cling-film
5. Refrigerate for 20 – 30 minutes.
6. As it refrigerates, dice the onion.
7. Cut the leek in half length-wise. Further cut each half again, chop.
8. Pour oil in a skillet, add the onion together with the leek.
9. Sauté for 5 minutes on medium temperature.
10. Add the frozen spinach continue to Sauté for more 5 minutes.
11. Turn off the heat.
12. Add seasoning stir frequently.
13. In a medium sized bowl, whisk the eggs, milk, and half and half until fully combined.
14. Grate the cheese.
15. Take out the pastry, divide into 2 pieces. Neatly roll out each of them ensure to make then larger than the pan bottom due to the need to cover them.
16. Make sure to line the pans with baking parchment and grease the sides with butter.
17. Place the crust pastry in.

18. With your hands, press the pastry down and to the sides.

19. With the back of your knife cut off the excess pastry.

20. Divide the filling into two equal halves and spread onto each pastry.

21. Pour the egg mixture over, top with cheese.

22. Proceed to bake in a preheated oven at 180° for 25 minutes.

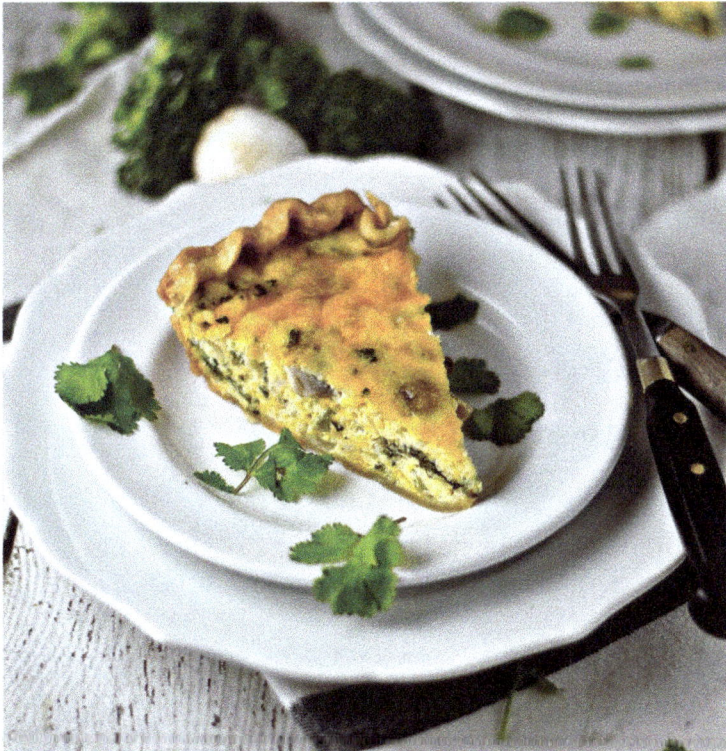

23. Serve and enjoy.

Artichoke tart

Cooked with spring onions and prosciutto, this artichoke tart is perfect for anyone. It utilizes range of ingredients and flavors topped with juicy tomatoes and roasted with roasted peppers.

Ingredients

- 2 tablespoon of roasted red pepper pesto
- 1 teaspoon of rosemary, optional
- 6 slices of prosciutto
- ½ cup of cheddar cheese (50g)
- 8 cherry tomatoes
- 1 puff pastry sheet
- ½ cup of green olives
- 2 spring onions
- 2 chili peppers
- 1 cup of artichoke hearts

Directions

1. Preheat your oven ready to 200°.
2. Roll out the pastry and cut in half.

3. Place both puff pastry sheets onto a baking tray lined with parchment paper.
4. Endeavor to ensure there is space in between the sheets.
5. Using a pizza cutter carefully cut out a rectangle ½ inch on both pastries from the edges.
6. Spread pesto over the pastry sheets.
7. Sprinkle cheese over and top each with the rest of the remaining ingredients.
8. Bake in the preheated oven for 12 minutes.
9. Serve and enjoy.

Chilaquiles Verde with baked tortilla chips

This recipe is Mexican by genesis fantastic for breakfast, lunch and dinner prepared with tortilla chips.

Ingredients

- 2 tablespoons of chopped cilantro
- ⅓ cup of crumbled Cotjia
- 2 teaspoons of extra-virgin olive oil
- 3 cups of salsa Verde
- 16 corn tortillas
- 4 fried eggs
- 1 avocado
- ½ teaspoon of sea salt
- 3 tablespoons of chopped red onion or green onion
- 2 tablespoons of extra-virgin olive oil
- 2 tablespoons of chopped fresh cilantro

Directions

1. Preheat your oven to 400°F.
2. Align two large baking sheets with parchment paper.

3. Brush the tortilla lightly with oil.
4. Stack and slice them into 8 wedges for all.
5. Arrange them evenly across the pans.
6. Sprinkle salt over all the pans.
7. Bake, swapping the pans on their racks every 5 minutes, until the chips are curling up at the edges in 10 minutes.
8. Warm 2 teaspoons of the olive oil in a large skillet over medium heat.
9. Add the salsa Verde once the pan is hot enough.
10. Lower the heat to simmer, then remove the skillet from the heat.
11. Stir in the tortilla chips with cilantro to coated all chips
12. Cover and let the rest until soft in 2 – 5 minutes.
13. Add the toppings.
14. Serve and enjoy.

Vegan mac and cheese

Ingredients

- 1 head of broccoli
- 3 teaspoons of apple cider vinegar
- 1 small yellow onion
- ½ teaspoon of garlic powder
- ½ teaspoon of onion powder
- ½ teaspoon of dry mustard powder
- Small pinch of red pepper flakes
- 3 cloves garlic, minced
- ⅔ cup of raw cashews
- 1 ½ tablespoons of avocado oil
- 8 ounces of whole-grain macaroni elbows
- 1 cup of water
- 1 cup of peeled and grated russet potato
- ½ teaspoon of salt
- ¼ cup of yeast

Directions

1. Boil salted water in a large pot. Place in the pasta and cook according to package instruction.

2. Drain, and transfer to a large serving bowl when not completely ready.
3. Warm oil over medium heat.
4. Add onion and a pinch of salt let cook, until the onion translucent in 5 minutes.
5. Add the grated potato, garlic powder, garlic, mustard powder, onion powder, salt and red pepper flakes stir to combine and cook for 1 minute.
6. Add cashews with water, stir to combine.
7. Simmer over reduced heat, stirring frequently for 5 – 8 minutes.
8. Pour mixture into a blender together with yeast and vinegar. Blend. For 2 minutes.
9. Taste and blend accordingly.
10. Transfer the sauce into the bowl of pasta. Stir to combine.
11. Serve soon enough and enjoy.

Almond sesame soda noodles with quick-pickled veggies

Ingredients

- 1 large cucumber
- 2 teaspoons of salt, divided
- 1 tablespoon sesame seeds
- ½ cup of unsalted almond butter
- Sriracha
- 1 small garlic clove, minced
- ¼ cup of freshly squeezed lime juice
- 2 tablespoons of tamari
- 8 ounces of soba noodles
- 2 teaspoons of raw honey
- 1 bunch of radishes
- 2 teaspoons toasted sesame oil
- ¼ cup water
- ¼ cup of rice vinegar
- 2 large zucchini

Directions

1. Start by cooking the noodles as per the package instruction, set aside after draining.
2. Combine cucumber with vinegar, radishes, and salt, let marinate for 10 minutes keep tossing.
3. In a smaller mixing bowl, combine garlic, almond butter, lime juice, honey, tamari, sesame oil and salt whisk to until blended. Place little water blend again briefly as required.
4. Place the sauce into the mixing bowl together with the soba noodles.
5. Add zucchini noodles toss to coated.
6. Put in serving dishes, top with quick-pickled veggies.
7. Garnish with sesame seeds.
8. Serve at room temperature.
9. Enjoy.

Broccolini almond pizza

Red sauce and mozzarella with blanched broccolini makes the perfect delicious pizza best for breakfast, lunch and dinner in less than 40 minutes.

Ingredients

- Red pepper flakes
- ¼ cup of sliced almonds
- ⅔ cup pizza sauce
- ½ cup of crumbled feta
- 1 batch easy whole wheat
- ½ pound of broccolini
- 1 teaspoon of extra-virgin olive oil
- 2 cups shredded low-moisture mozzarella cheese

Directions

1. Preheat your oven to 500°F.
2. Spread marinara sauce evenly over the pizza.
3. Pour the mozzarella, feta and almonds over the pizza.
4. Boil water in a saucepan. Trim the broccolini.
5. Toss in the broccolini, let boil for 1 minute.
6. Drain and pat dry.

7. Then, toss again with 1 teaspoon of olive oil to coat lightly.
8. Assemble the broccolini over the pizza.
9. Sprinkle the almonds on top.
10. Bake pizza on the top rack until golden in 12 minutes.
11. Transfer to a cutting board
12. Sprinkle with red pepper flakes.
13. Slice, serve and enjoy.

Hummus quesadillas

Unlike with cheese, this quesadilla is typically prepared with hummus delicious enough to keep you hooked the whole day. it is gluten and dairy free vegan healthy recipe.

Ingredients

- One 8-inch whole grain tortilla
- ⅓ cup hummus
- Fillings of your choice
- Extra-virgin olive oil

Directions

1. Begin by spreading hummus over the tortilla.
2. Lightly cover one-half of the tortilla with fillings.
3. Fold the blank half over. Make as needed.
4. Warm a medium skillet over medium heat.
5. Place folded quesadilla(s) in the pan.
6. Warm lower sides briefly. Brush with olive oil, let cook in the pan for 2 minutes. Repeat this step for the other side. Continue to cook until all sides turn golden.
7. Transfer to a cutting board let rest briefly.
8. Slice into 3 wedges.
9. Serve and enjoy.

Lentil baked ziti

Ingredients

- Basil leaves
- 2 cloves garlic, minced
- 1 ¼ cups of regular brown lentils
- 3 cups of water
- ¼ teaspoon of salt
- Freshly ground black pepper
- Pinch of red pepper flakes
- 1 red onion
- 23.5 ounces of Marinara
- 1 tablespoon of olive oil
- 8 ounces of grated mozzarella cheese
- 1 cup cottage cheese
- 12 ounces of whole grain ziti

Directions

1. Warm olive oil until shimmering without smoke in a large saucepan.
2. Add onion and salt cook until onions turn translucent in 5 minutes
3. Add garlic let cook for 30 seconds or until fragrant.

4. Add lentils with water, stir to combine.

5. Increase the heat to high, then lower after 25 minutes, let simmer over low heat for 15 minutes.

6. Drain out excess water. Set aside.

7. Preheat your oven to 350°F.

8. Place salted water to boil in a large saucepan. Place the pasta to cook as instructed on the package.

9. Drain excess water return to the saucepan.

10. Add the lentils to the pasta.

11. Add cheese, leave some for later.

12. Season to taste with salt and freshly ground black pepper.

13. Pour to the baking dish evenly spread the sauce to coat.

14. Pour the lentil together with pasta into the baker, spread. Dollop cheese over the mixture.

15. Drizzle the balance over the dish.

16. Cover the baker tightly. Bake for 30 minutes.

17. Continue baking when uncovered at higher heat until golden.

18. Remove the baker from the oven let it cool for 10 minutes.

19. Sprinkle with basil.

20. Serve and enjoy.

Spring veggie stir fry

This meal gets ready only in 20 minutes served with rice and any protein source.

Ingredients

- 2 teaspoons of arrowroot starch
- 3 medium carrots
- 1 tablespoon of grated fresh ginger
- ½ bunch of thin asparagus
- Pinch of salt
- 1 large clove garlic minced
- ½ teaspoon of crushed red pepper
- 1 tablespoon of coconut oil
- ¼ cup of Soy Sauce
- 2 tablespoons of Wildflower Honey
- 1 small red onion

Directions

1. Combine soy sauce, cornstarch, honey, garlic, ginger, and red pepper flakes. Whisk until blended.

2. Warm oil over medium temperature until shimmering without smoke.

3. Add onion together with carrots and salt.

4. Increase the heat to high cook, stirring frequently to soften onions in 5 minutes.

5. Add asparagus let cook for 3 minutes or until carrots begin to caramelize on the edges.

6. Pour in the prepared sauce and cook for 1 minute or until thick.

7. Serve and enjoy.

Sweet potato and black bean tacos

Beans could not be any more delicious with avocado pepitas dip. The recipe takes only 30 minutes to prepare this vegan meal for lunch or dinner or even breakfast.

Ingredients

- Olive oil
- Salt
- Ground cumin
- Crumbled feta
- 2 cans of black beans
- Water
- 2 avocado pitted
- 1 cup of lightly packed fresh cilantro
- 2 pounds of sweet potatoes
- ½ cup pepitas
- 1 small jalapeño
- Ground black pepper
- 2 cloves garlic
- ¼ teaspoon of cayenne pepper
- 1 teaspoon of cherry vinegar
- 2 tablespoons lime juice

- 1 yellow onion
- 10 small corn tortillas
- ¼ teaspoon of chili powder

Directions

1. Preheat the oven to 425°F.
2. Align a large baking sheet with parchment paper.
3. Toss potatoes with olive oil, cayenne pepper, and salt.
4. Organize in a single layer bake for 30 – 40 minutes toss halfway, until tender.
5. Warm the olive oil in a large saucepan over medium heat.
6. Add onions sprinkled with salt let cook for 5 – 8 minutes until onions turn translucent.
7. Add cumin together with the chili powder pour beans and water after 1 minute. Simmer over low heat covered.
8. Smash some of the beans then stir in the vinegar, season with salt and pepper.
9. Toast pepitas in a skillet over medium heat for 5 minutes. Transfer to a bowl, set aside.
10. Place avocado flesh into a food processor with jalapeño, cilantro, garlic, lime juice, water and salt. Blend until smooth.
11. Add the pepitas, process till they are chopped.
12. Taste and season accordingly. Keep in a small bowl.
13. Warm the tortillas.
14. Spread black beans down the middle of each tortilla.

15. Top with bit of sweet potatoes and avocado dip.

16. Garnish with feta and pepitas.

17. Serve and enjoy.

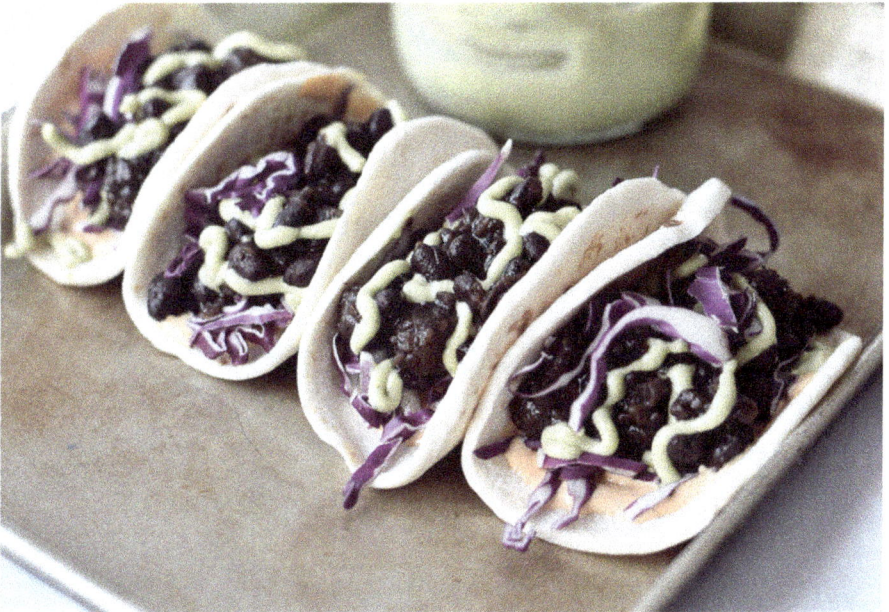

Vegan BLT sandwich

This tasty vegan sandwich is prepared with variety of vegetable; tomatoes, avocado, and coconut bacon. It is quite classic on the Mediterranean Sea diet menu for lunch and dinner in 12 minutes.

Ingredients

- 1 medium ripe avocado
- Salt
- Freshly ground black pepper
- Several small leaves of romaine
- ¼ cup of coconut bacon
- 1 medium ripe red tomato
- 2 slices of eureka

Instruction

1. Toast bread to your liking.
2. Scoop the avocado flesh into a bowl with a pinch of salt.
3. Mash the avocado with fork, till smooth.
4. Spread the bread with avocado.
5. Spread coconut bacon heavily on one piece of toast.
6. Press into the avocado to stick.

7. Slice the tomato into slices.

8. Top the bacon-covered toast with slices of tomato.

9. Sprinkle with black pepper.

10. Top tomato with lettuce and the other bread on top, avocado side down.

11. Enjoy the bites.

Vegan spaghetti alla puttanesca

If you are seeking for an ultimate super fresh taste, then seek no more, vegan spaghetti alla puttanesca prepared with pantry staple is a delicious vegan meal.

Ingredients

- 1 tablespoon of caper brine
- 3 cloves garlic, minced
- ½ cup chopped parsley leaves
- 1 tablespoon of olive oil
- 8 ounces of whole grain spaghetti
- ⅓ cup of chopped Kalamata olives
- Freshly ground black pepper
- ¼ teaspoon of red pepper flakes
- 1 large can of chunky tomato sauce
- ⅓ cup of capers
- Salt
- 1 tablespoon of Kalamata olive brine

Directions

1. Combine tomato sauce, olive bring, capers, olives, caper brine, garlic, and red pepper flakes in a saucepan.

2. Cook over high heat, then reduce heat to simmer, in 20 minute, keep stirring frequently.

3. Remove from heat, stir in olive oil and chopped parsley season with ground black pepper and salt.

4. As the sauce is cooking, place salted water in a large saucepan, cook as directed on the package.

5. Drain and return it to the pot.

6. Pour sauce over the pasta, stir gently to combine.

7. Place into bowls, top each bowl with a light sprinkle of parsley.

8. Serve immediately and enjoy.

Zucchini noodles with basil pumpkin

Ingredients

- ½ cup of pepitas
- Salt
- 1 garlic clove
- 2 cups of packed fresh basil leaves
- ⅓ cup of olive oil
- 2 teaspoons of red wine vinegar
- Pinch of red pepper flakes
- 3 large zucchini
- ½ small yellow onion
- Fresh basil leaves
- 1 pint of cherry tomatoes

Instruction

1. In a food processor, combine garlic, onion, toasted pepitas, basil, olive oil, vinegar and red pepper flakes.
2. Blend until smooth, season with salt.
3. Toss zucchini with pesto until coated, season with salt.
4. Transfer to a large platter.
5. Sprinkle with the cherry tomatoes.
6. Serve and enjoy.

Better broccoli casserole

This recipe takes another twist of roasted broccoli, with creamy quinoa and garlicky whole grain bread crumbs along with cheddar cheese. This undeniably healthy recipe is an amazing choice for breakfast or dinner.

Ingredients

- 1 slice of whole wheat bread
- 1 clove garlic minced
- 2 cups of vegetable broth or water
- Freshly ground black pepper
- ¾ teaspoon of salt
- ¼ teaspoon of red pepper flakes
- 1 cup of quinoa
- 8 ounces of freshly grated cheddar cheese
- 1 cup of low-fat milk
- 2 tablespoons of olive oil
- ½ tablespoon of butter
- 16 ounces of broccoli florets

Directions

1. Preheat oven to 400 °F.
2. Line a large baking sheet with parchment paper
3. Boil water in a medium sized saucepan.
4. Add quinoa, reduce heat to let simmer uncovered for 18 – 20 minutes.
5. Remove and steam for 10 minutes when covered.
6. Slice large broccoli to small pieces.
7. Move to baking sheet, toss with olive oil, until coated.
8. Arrange in a single layer then Sprinkle with salt.
9. Bake for 20 minutes, until tender.
10. Toss bread and place in a food processor. Process until broken into crumbs.
11. Melt butter in a small pan over medium heat.
12. Add garlic cook until fragrant.
13. Add the bread crumbs cook for 3 minutes keep aside.
14. Over low heat add salt, pepper and red pepper flakes to the pot of quinoa make sure to stir to combine.
15. Add cheese to the pot with milk stir to blend.
16. Pour mixture in a dish, top with roasted broccoli. Stir.
17. Sprinkle the casserole with cheese and breadcrumbs on top.
18. Bake while uncovered for 25 minutes.
19. Cool, serve and enjoy.

Spinach pasta with roasted broccoli and bell pepper

The vegetables are tossed with flavorful balsamic sauce and massively loaded with vegetables; spinach pasta. It is gluten free and vegan for a complete meal.

Ingredients

- Freshly ground black pepper
- 1 red bell pepper
- 2 tablespoons of balsamic vinegar
- Salt
- 1 shallot bulb.
- ¼ teaspoon of red pepper flakes
- 2 cloves garlic, pressed or minced
- 1 large bunch of broccoli
- 12 ounces of baby spinach
- 8 ounces of spaghetti
- 4 tablespoon of olive oil
- 1 tablespoon of lemon juice

Directions

1. Preheat your oven to 400°F.
2. Move broccoli florets with bell pepper to the baking sheet.
3. Drizzle with olive oil, toss to coated in oil.
4. Sprinkle with salt, then organize the vegetables in an even layer, bake until the broccoli is tender in 25 minutes.
5. Place salted water in a large pot, boil.
6. Cook past as directed on the package.
7. Drain and reserve some pasta water.
8. Get large pan, sauté over medium heat, place olive oil to shimmer.
9. Add shallot, salt and red pepper flakes cook for 5 minutes till shallots are translucent.
10. Add garlic let cook 20 seconds and spinach to wilt, repeat for all spinach.
11. Pour in balsamic vinegar take pot off heat source.
12. Combine roasted vegetables with cooked pasta and spinach mixture.
13. Add lemon juice, olive oil.
14. Drizzle with pasta cooking water, toss.
15. Season to taste with salt and freshly ground black pepper.
16. Serve and enjoy.

Spaghetti squash burrito bowls

Ingredients

- Salt
- Freshly ground black pepper
- 2 cups purple cabbage
- Fresh lime juice
- 1 can of black beans.
- 1 red bell pepper, chopped
- 2 tablespoons olive oil
- Fresh cilantro
- ¾ cup of mild salsa Verde
- 1 medium garlic clove
- 2 medium spaghetti squash
- 1 ripe avocado, diced
- ⅓ cup chopped green onions

Directions

1. Preheat the oven to 400°F.
2. Prepare a large baking sheet with parchment paper.
3. Drizzle spaghetti squash with olive oil, rub all over each of the halves.

4. Sprinkle the insides of the squash with freshly ground black pepper, salt.
5. Roast for 45 minutes, until easily pierced through.
6. In a medium mixing bowl, combine black beans, cabbage, bell pepper, cilantro, green onion, olive oil, lime juice, and salt. Toss. Keep aside as it marinates.
7. In a separate bowl of a blender, combine cilantro, salsa Verde, avocado, lime juice, and garlic. Blend until smooth.
8. Divide the slaw into spaghetti squash
9. Add avocado salsa Verde.
10. Sprinkle again with pepper and cilantro.
11. Serve and enjoy.

Pasta primavera

This pasta features a bunch of healthy roasted Mediterranean vegetables for a powerful dish. Season it with thyme and oregano for a tastier recipe.

Ingredients

- 8 oz. of grape tomatoes halved
- 3 carrots peeled and cut into short sticks
- Black pepper
- 1 red bell pepper cored and sliced into thin sticks
- ½ cup parmesan cheese more to your liking
- Zest of 1 large lemon
- 1 yellow or orange bell pepper cored and sliced
- 1 red onion halved and sliced
- 3 large garlic cloves minced
- 1 tablespoons of dried oregano more for later
- 2 zucchini halved length-wise and sliced
- 1 ½ teaspoon of fresh thyme more for later
- Kosher salt
- Extra virgin olive oil
- 2 yellow squash halved length-wise and sliced
- 12 ounces of short pasta

Directions

1. Heat your oven to 450°F.
2. Place the vegetables in a large mixing bowl at once.
3. Add garlic, oregano, and thyme.
4. Season with a pinch of kosher salt and black pepper.
5. Drizzle a good amount of extra virgin olive oil. Toss.
6. Move the vegetables to a large sheet pan.
7. Spread them out well.
8. Then, roast in heated oven for 20 minutes.
9. Cook pasta in salted boiling water as per the Directions on the package.
10. Drain and excess water reserving some for later.
11. Move pasta to a large bowl.
12. Season with salt and pepper and little oregano and fresh thyme.
13. Place in the vegetables.
14. Now, add the tomatoes together with the lemon zest.
15. Add a bit of the reserved pasta cooking water with a bit of extra virgin olive oil. Toss.
16. Sprinkle with parmesan cheese.
17. Serve and enjoy immediately.

Lemon broccoli pesto pasta

Prepared with a splash of lemon, this lemon pesto pasta is loaded with other tasty flavors and herbs for a perfect Mediterranean taste.

Ingredients

- Freshly cracked black pepper
- 1 lb.. short pasta
- 6 tablespoons of pine nuts, lightly toasted
- 2 cups of packed fresh basil leaves
- Kosher salt
- Zest and juice of 2 lemons
- 3 cups of grated Parmesan cheese
- 12 ounces of frozen broccoli
- 1 cup of extra virgin olive oil

Directions

1. Boil water in a large pot and salt.
2. Add the broccoli and cook until crisp tender in 4 minutes.
3. Transfer the broccoli to a large bowl of ice water. Reserve and cooking water for later.
4. Drain and dry on a paper towel.

5. In the bowl of a food processor, combine the broccoli, 4 tablespoon of the pine nuts, basil leaves, Parmesan, and lemon zest and juice.
6. Process until combined.
7. Scrape down the sides of the bowl, run the processor again.
8. Slowly stream in the extra virgin olive oil as the processor is still running.
9. Season with salt and pepper.
10. Bring the same pot of water back to a boil.
11. Then, add the pasta, cook as per the package Directions.
12. Drain the pasta and reserve some water.
13. Return the drained pasta to the pot over medium heat.
14. Add 1 cup of the Parmesan cheese with the reserved pasta water, let cook as you stir constantly for 1 minute.
15. Remove from heat source, then add half of the broccoli pesto. Toss.
16. Transfer the pasta to a large serving bowl.
17. Top with the remaining Parmesan cheese and pine nuts or lemon juice.
18. Serve and enjoy when garnished with basil leaves.

Stuffed tomato recipe

The stuffed tomato recipe derives its aromatic flavor from garlic and onions among other tasty spices and it makes a perfect Mediterranean Sea diet stuffed recipe.

Ingredients

- 6 large tomatoes
- 1 large red onion halved, minced
- 1 teaspoon of ground cumin
- 4 garlic cloves, minced
- ½ lb.. lean ground beef
- Kosher salt and black pepper
- ½ teaspoon of allspice
- Extra virgin olive oil
- 2 cups of canned crushed tomatoes
- ½ cup of white wine
- ½ teaspoon of ground nutmeg
- ¼ cup of water
- ½ cup long grain rice
- ¾ teaspoon of dried oregano
- 1 cup of chopped fresh parsley
- ½ cup of chopped fresh spearmint

Directions

1. Place the rice in a bowl and cover with water.

2. Soak for 20 minutes until it is easy to break one grain of rice between your fingertips.

3. Drain any excess water.

4. Preheat your oven to 375°F.

5. Place a large skillet over medium-high heat.

6. Add ⅓ cup of extra virgin olive oil let heat until just shimmering but with no smoke.

7. Add chopped onions together with the garlic, toss until fragrant.

8. Add the ground meat, season with salt, pepper, cumin, oregano, nutmeg, and allspice and let cook for 5 minutes or until fully browned.

9. Add drained rice it to the meat mixture in the skillet.

10. Add crushed tomatoes together with the white wine and water.

11. Bring the saucy mixture to a boil, lower the heat let simmer for 10 minutes.

12. Stir in the fresh herbs.

13. Season with kosher salt.

14. Cut tomato tops and keep the tops aside.

15. Loosen the tomatoes with a knife by going around the edges of the tomato.

16. Scoop out the tomato flesh and chop the flesh into large pieces, keep for later.

17. Prepare a baking pan by oiling the bottom with extra virgin olive oil.
18. Spread the chopped tomato flesh and sliced onion at the bottom of the baking dish.
19. Add the chopped tomato flesh together with the sliced onion to make a bed for the stuffed tomatoes.
20. Spoon the saucy meat and rice mixture into the empty tomato shells.
21. Organize the stuffed tomatoes in the prepared baking dish.
22. Cover with the reserved tops.
23. From one of the corners of your baking dish, carefully pour ¾ cup of water.
24. Add a little pinch of salt and a generous drizzle of extra virgin olive oil on top.
25. Cover the baking dish with foil let bake in heated oven for 45 minutes.
26. Let cook uncovered for more 45 minutes.
27. Let cool.
28. Serve and enjoy.

Classic tiramisu

This mighty classic tiramisu features ladyfingers dipped in espresso together with Kahlua layer of a mascarpone custard fluffy with tasty cream.

Ingredients

- 8 ounces of mascarpone cheese at room temperature
- ½ cup plus 2 tablespoons of Kahlua liqueur
- 1 teaspoon of vanilla extract
- 3 eggs
- ½ cup of granulated sugar divided
- 1 cup of boiling water
- 1 7- ounce package of Savoiardi cookies
- Cocoa powder
- 4 cups of whipping cream
- 6 tablespoons of Instant espresso powder

Directions

1. Bring 1 cup of water to a boil.
2. Pour into a shallow bowl.

3. Mix in the espresso powder and ½ cup of the Kahlua liqueur. Set aside to cool.

4. Separate the egg yolks from the whites, make sure to save the whites.

5. Add the yolks to a small, heat proof bowl that fits snugly over another saucepan filled with about 2 inches of water.

6. Let the water simmer gently and top with the bowl of egg yolks.

7. Add ¼ cup of sugar to the egg yolks, use a hand mixer to beat the eggs on medium speed over the simmering water for 5 minutes until the mixtures is creamy and light yellow.

8. Remove the bowl from the heat, let cool.

9. In another large bowl, add the whipping cream, remaining ¼ cup of sugar, 2 tablespoons Kahlua and the vanilla, beat until stiff peaks form.

10. Shift the cooled egg yolk mixture to a large bowl.

11. Add the mascarpone to the egg yolk mixture and blend until smooth.

12. Gently fold the whipping cream into the egg yolk mixture with a large spatula.

13. Toss the ladyfingers in the espresso mixture and arrange half of them in a single layer in the bottom of a pan.

14. Spread half of the whipped cream mixture over the ladyfingers.

15. Let soak the remaining ladyfingers 3 at a time to create another layer and top with the remaining whip cream mixture and spread equally over the top.

16. Cover with plastic wrap and refrigerate for at 8 hours up to 48 hours.

17. Run a knife along the inside of the pan and cut into squares.

18. Dust the servings with cocoa powder and serve.

19. Enjoy.

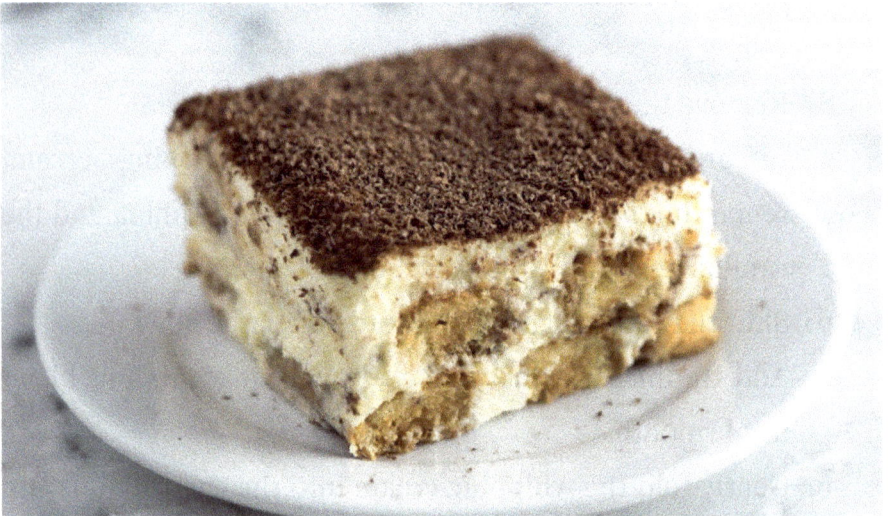

Za'atar manaquish recipe

The eastern Mediterranean region makes this recipe as their favorite featuring vegetables and tasty and aromatic spices.

Ingredients

- 1 cup of lukewarm water
- Radish
- ½ cup of extra virgin olive oil
- ½ teaspoon of sugar
- 3 cups unbleached all-purpose flour,
- Feta cheese
- Cucumbers
- 1 tsp salt
- 2 tablespoons of extra virgin olive oil
- 8 tablespoons of quality Za'atar spice
- 2 ¼ teaspoons of active dry yeast
- Tomatoes
- Olives

Directions

1. Preheat your oven to 400°F. Place a large baking sheet in oven while heating

2. In a small bowl, combine water, sugar and yeast. Keep for 10 minutes to let foam.

3. In another separate large mixing bowl, combine flour together with salt, and olive oil.

4. Work the mixture with your hands.

5. Make a well in the middle and pour in the yeast and water mixture. Stir until soft dough forms.

6. Turn dough onto a lightly floured surface and knead for 10 minutes or until dough is elastic, smooth.

7. Form dough into a ball and place in a lightly oiled mixing bowl.

8. Cover with damp cloth and place in a warm spot and let rise for 2 hours.

9. Punch dough down. Knead briefly and form into 8 small balls.

10. Organize on lightly floured surface, cover again and leave to rise for more 30 minutes.

11. Next, mix together the za'atar spice and olive oil in a bowl.

12. Lightly oil the heated baking sheet and set close.

13. Flatten the dough into small discs.

14. Make indentations in discs.

15. Add 1 tablespoon of za'atar topping in the middle of each disc, leave a narrow boarder around.
16. Organize the discs in prepared oiled baking sheet.
17. Bake in the preheated-oven for 8 minutes.
18. Remove from heat and let sit for 5 minutes.
19. Topping will dry and settle into dough.
20. Serve za'atar manaquish warm with assorted vegetables.
21. Enjoy.

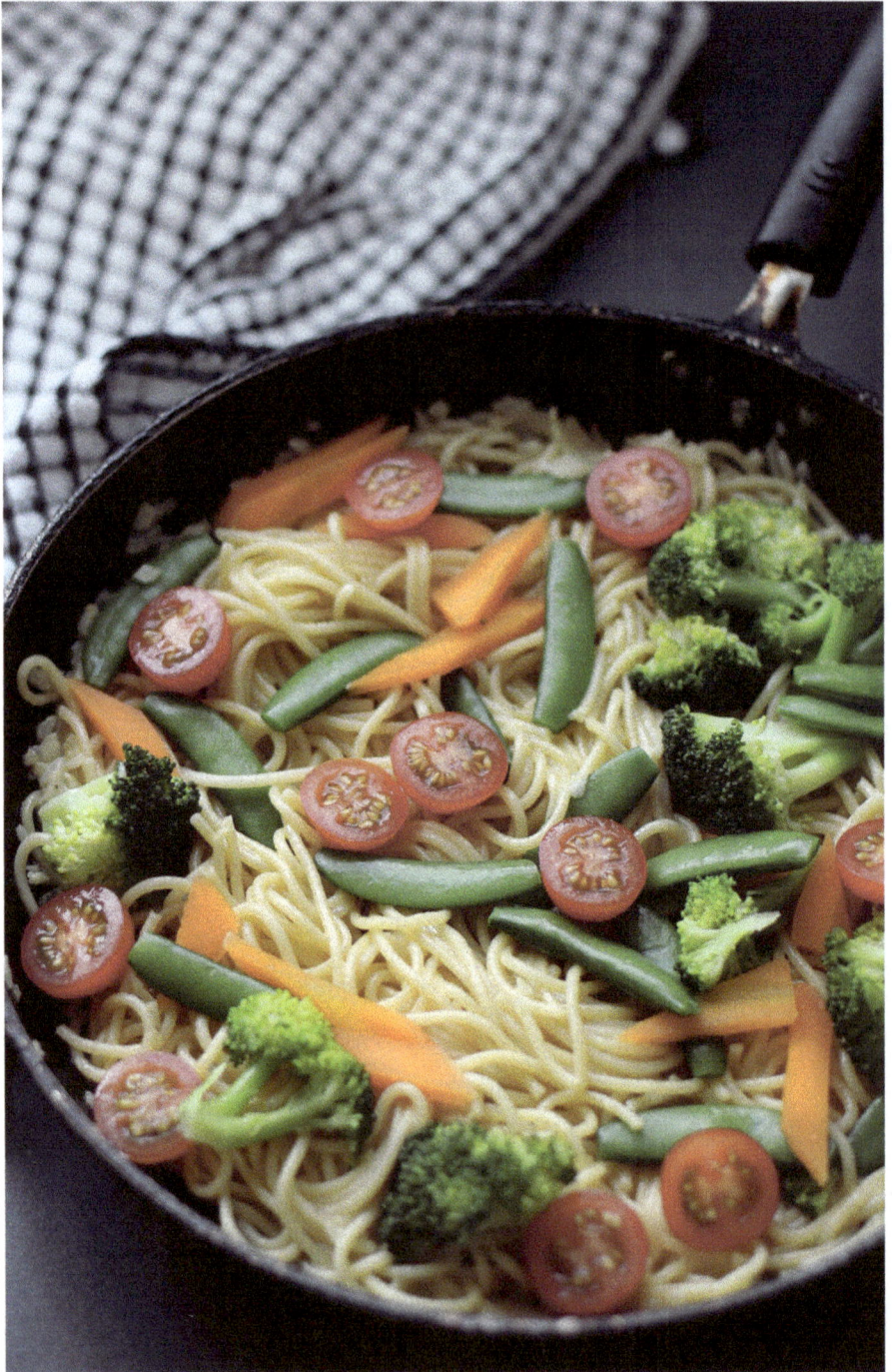

www.ingramcontent.com/pod-product-compliance
Lightning Source LLC
Chambersburg PA
CBHW050746030426
42336CB00012B/1679